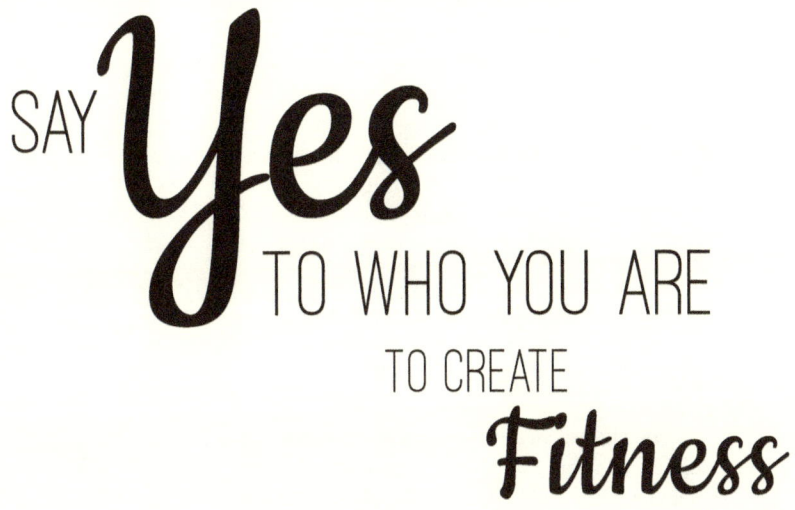

SAY Yes TO WHO YOU ARE TO CREATE Fitness

TRICIA GUNBERG

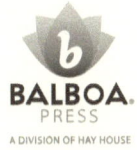

BALBOA
PRESS
A DIVISION OF HAY HOUSE

Balboa Press books may be ordered through booksellers or by contacting:

Balboa Press
A Division of Hay House
1663 Liberty Drive
Bloomington, IN 47403
www.balboapress.com
1 (877) 407-4847

Because of the dynamic nature of the Internet, any web addresses or links contained in this book may have changed since publication and may no longer be valid. The views expressed in this work are solely those of the author and do not necessarily reflect the views of the publisher, and the publisher hereby disclaims any responsibility for them.

The author of this book does not dispense medical advice or prescribe the use of any technique as a form of treatment for physical, emotional, or medical problems without the advice of a physician, either directly or indirectly. The intent of the author is only to offer information of a general nature to help you in your quest for emotional and spiritual well-being. In the event you use any of the information in this book for yourself, which is your constitutional right, the author and the publisher assume no responsibility for your actions.

Any people depicted in stock imagery provided by Thinkstock are models, and such images are being used for illustrative purposes only. Certain stock imagery © Thinkstock.

Print information available on the last page.

ISBN: 978-1-5043-5847-7 (sc)
ISBN: 978-1-5043-5849-1 (hc)
ISBN: 978-1-5043-5848-4 (e)

Library of Congress Control Number: 2016908508

Balboa Press rev. date: 07/26/2016

CONTENTS

DEDICATION

I dedicate this book to the person who first encouraged my writing.
He continues to send me reminders to keep at the art. Thank you dad
for seeing something in me so long ago that I could not see in myself.
Also, thank you for the continued encouragement. It adds the joyful
prodding I need and it always comes when I need it most.

With love, deep understanding, a side of sauerkraut and a dash of
fresh garlic,

Your daughter

ACKNOWLEDGEMENTS

To put one name on the cover of this book seems so unfair and not completely truthful. Yes, I did write it but not without the support of so many. First to my dear husband Nathan, wow, that agreement to take 6 months off to write seems like a joke doesn't it? Thank you so much for allowing me all the time I needed to explore my writing and spirituality. Also, for listening to me ramble on about my latest discovery and for all your hours of correcting my spelling. As a heads up: this is just the beginning so I hope you're ready for more. Secondly, to my brilliant friends Jan Peiper and Cheryl Steimel, your sharp eyes and professional guidance in the editing (Ugh!) process made it feasible. Mahalo to my friends Malia Durbano and Annie Kelleher who lead by excellent example. Lastly, to my family, for their support and understanding. They have always been there for me no matter what I have gotten myself into, so I am glad to have the opportunity to thank them. Special thanks to my niece Cassie Servi who knows my artistic side and for graciously sharing hers with me.

INTRODUCTION

What it comes down to is choices. Do you realize your life is just a series of choices, big and small? Making the choices for your greatest and highest good is the key. This information is presented to you so you can recognize your true self and make choices accordingly. Are you ready to say "yes" to who you really are and find more health? Are you ready to see these truths that will serve as building blocks to your success?

My personal struggles propelled me to question. Why am I sad? Why do I have elevated blood pressure? Why do I continue to make unhealthy choices? Why am I taking a pill instead of finding the cause? All of the knowledge I have gained was purely from a selfish stand point. I understand now, that life requires us to be selfish in order to become selfless. Like oxygen on an airplane- serving yourself first is necessary. Learning about the body-mind connection and understanding myself and clients through numerology answered so many of my questions. Both of these have now become a welcomed way of life. While I 'accidently' blended this knowledge with my background to support my clients and myself, the resulting program I pioneered is no accident.

If I do not continue to work to understand myself and learn how to work with my numerology, I would continue to be ill and feel overwhelmed. The daily activities I now engage in feed my soul. Having yoga, swimming, cooking, and art, in my life are the same as water, oxygen and food- these important elements I would not have been aware of if it was not for numerology.

It is my hope you are set free by the ideas you find here. That you will feel the freedom to explore who you are and the freedom to feel good about what you discover about yourself.

SAY *Yes*

TO WHO YOU ARE

TO CREATE

Fitness

TRICIA GUNBERG

CHAPTER 1

Why We Avoid Exercise
and what we can do about it

"We all bounce around between the extremes of codependency and control, until we remember our 'divineness' and become centered. Our goal is to recognize our issues through our challenges. Once we recognize our patterns, we can alter them to achieve better health and well-being."
MICHAEL BRILL

You know when you are not quite ready to do something and then along comes a solution? Here it is. You were thinking about getting fit and you found this book.

What is the reason we avoid exercise? My clients provide many excuses as to why they cannot add healthy choices to their lives. By sighting lack of time, commitment to family, and the need to work with so much conviction, they almost convince me. A few times, I swear the person thought I said "Would you like some crack cocaine?" instead of, "Would you consider yoga? I think it would really help you." What is the resistance? I wondered this time and time again. I also wondered why so many avoid the thing that could help them the most.

By discovering some of the reasons people avoid exercise, I began to look at those excuses in a different way. The reasons are usually deeply hidden; you may not even realize some of these. Are any of them you? Do they sound like an acceptable reason to avoid exercise?

- You would rather be doing something that would change the way you look instantaneously. Like apply make-up or wear slimming clothes.
- You would rather be tending to other people's needs and have a hard time justifying spending time on yourself.
- You would rather be out and about creating things and socializing.
- You would rather being empowering someone to add fitness to their lives.
- You would rather do anything else than having a predictable approach to anything.
- You would rather be planning a gala or event for fit people.
- You would rather be teaching others fitness.
- You would rather be making money or working, as you see no financial gain in your health.
- You are here to save the world so you get a bit tired sometimes.

These are reasons and good ones too; saving time, helping others, supporting loved ones, making money and saving the world. It is no wonder with reasons like these so many of us go without a fitness routine.

If we take these same ideas and twist them just a little bit we get this:

- You want to look good, you just don't want to spend a lot of time doing it.
- You will create MORE energy, more attentiveness, and more love. AND there will be *more* of you to share with others *if* you take care of yourself.
- What you have yet to learn is fitness and health is social and can have a creative aspect. You can hang-out with others in healthier situations and still enJOY yourself.
- You can clearly see a step-by-step process others can apply, but you overlook it for yourself.
- You do not know a fitness routine does not have to be routine. You can make it fun and unpredictable and still accomplish your fitness goals.
- You reserve your love for others and only apply a little to yourself. When you realize the love you give yourself will be multiplied, you will have three times more to give others.
- You miss workouts because you have not found something that works for you.
- Seeing no immediate gain to staying fit can thwart your efforts. You are a worthy cause and as soon as you realize this you will not miss a work out again.
- You need to channel your energy into "fitness with a cause." Build your muscle while you build a better world.

I will show you how to make a program out of this but give me a minute while I dispel two other factors: time and resistance. A big fat strawberry to the concept of time having anything to do with the inability to stick with a fitness program. Lack of time is an excuse, a very bad one, at that. We all have the same amount of time, the same 24 hours in a day, yet some of us are fit and some of us are not. Time is not an excuse because we all have the same amount and we are able to choose how we spend it. The choices we have made create the illusion of not having enough time. Do you spend your time the same way as your neighbor? You think this is a ridiculous question, but why do you spend your time in a way that prevents exercise and staying fit? Time feels like a valid excuse but it is not the reason you avoid exercise.

There is part of you resisting things that are good for you. It is odd for humans to have this ability. Many refer to this part of ourselves as ego and defining it as, "edging good out" or "edging god out." When I first started watching my thoughts, I had all sorts of names for the part of me that tells me untruths about myself. Not nice names either. In realizing it is never a good idea to be angry at one's self, I concentrated on the part of me which helps make loving decisions and refer to it as 'my higher self'. This book will give you ways to access to your higher self and be less engaged with your ego self.

Your life is a series of choices, big and small. You can gain the wisdom you need to make the choices for your greatest and highest good. From the type of exercise that fits you best, to the duration and frequency. There is more to you than meets the eye. Your greatest strengths can become your greatest weaknesses if they go unattended. Your strengths can become your greatest assets. By delving into the metaphysical, just a bit, the truth about you will be revealed. This information is presented to you so you can recognize your true self, and to say "yes" to who you really are. Presented in the form of attributes, these truths will serve as building blocks to your success.

What if I told you these same reasons we avoid exercise, which were derived from numerology, also have a solution derived from numerology? There is a reason behind your resistance to creating and staying with a fitness program, I found these reasons through numerology. I also found the solution (positive aspects) through numerology as well. Your numerology chart refers to several numbers based on your birth name and your date of birth. Some of the numbers in the chart provide an overview on your life, while other numbers get a bit more specific. Any one of these numbers in your chart could be described at length. The most commonly known is the Life Purpose Number or Life Path Number. This is the number that is calculated by adding the digits of your birthday. The Life Path number is renamed in my system as the Health and Wellness Path number.

Numerology is a system that describes a relationship between numbers and things. It is a code, like musical notes or letters of a language. Numbers contain energy and when applied to things, provide meaning. They speak to you, much like music, at the soul level. When you align yourself with the numbers in your cart, amazing things happen.

- It provides you with information to help you set meaningful intention and awareness of appropriate goals. Most important, it offers support with your goals.
- This energy is there for us to tap into. Similar to how we can tap into our dreams, we can tap into numbers.

- Just as we could use our dreams to solve our daily problems, shed light on our fears and get inspiration, we can do the same with numerology.
- It beckons us to come into harmony with the true nature of ourselves.
- Numerology aids you in honoring self.
- This natural process will empower you to take notice of your life.
- Through finding meaning and fulfillment in who you are, you can accomplish anything.
- It provides you with information to discover your own truth.
- Ways of coming closer to your Soul and all aspects of self.
- Gaining awareness of what constitutes 'you'. Body awareness is the best type of awareness to transform and extend the understanding you have of yourself. It is said your body is your connection to Spirit and Soul.

Consider numerology as energy in the form of information. As in dreamtime, numerology's only power is when we use it to our advantage. Dream interpretation can be quite complicated, to the point where people are in complete denial of its power. When we cannot clearly see information in a dream, we think it is of no value. In truth, this is correct. The power comes from the interpretation and application.

One of the systems I use early on, to generate numerology readings, is from *The Life You Were Born to Live*. In it, the author, Dan Millman traces numerology back to ancient Greece. As to how the Life Purpose System works, Dan Millan states, "I can't rationally explain how...I can only know, based on empirical testing, that the system works- that it can bring lives into focus."

By assigning numeric values to letters A, J, S = 1, B, K, T = 2 and so on, then totaling the numbers until the outcome of a single digit, provides its meaning. You may already be acquainted with some of these: 1is being "first" or striving to be number one, 2 represents balance (ying/yang, dark/light), and the number 8 is abundance (infinity symbol standing up).

To find the energy of any word, we find the value for each letter then add the numbers together until we get a single digit. For example lets us use my name as an example. My first name has the number value of 6. This means on my best day I am: cheerful, loving, and energetic.

On an off day I am: hypocritical, easily stressed or restless. For that is the energy of the six. Here is how we calculate the name Tricia:

T=2　**R**=9　**I**=9　**C**=3　**I**=9　**A**=1
2　+　9　+　9　+　3　+　9　+　1 = 33
We continue adding the 33 to get a single digit.
3 + 3 = 6

Your birthdate is already in numerical form so we add it until it becomes a single digit. This is your birth path or Life Purpose Number. This can reveal so much about your true self. My birthdate is August 4, 1969. Reducing them to single digit looks like this:

8 + 4 + 1 + 9 + 6 + 9 = 37
37 is added again:
3 + 7 = 10
10 is added again:
1 + 0 = 1

My Life Path is 1. A brief description of this Life Path according to Dan Millman is: "here to work through issues of creativity while learning to trust the wise and beautiful spirit with-in themselves and others, and to apply their inner gifts to create more harmony in the world." Since reading that statement I have been discovering what it means for me. So far it has been an exciting journey.

Before we get into how to create your fitness based on your numerology I want to give you general meanings for each of the numbers. The characteristics of these numbers are important because, as I explained, they are characteristics of you.

The reality is you need to understand when an attribute is getting out of control. If knowing the less peasant parts, or challenges, of your attributes appeals to you, add those too. Michael Brill does an excellent job in his book *Numerology for Healing* if you want to know the challenges of your numerology as they relate to illnesses.

Here are a list of attributes/characteristics for each number for you to start exploring. Every attribute has a not so positive side to them. The number two is a good example of this as one of its attributes is sensitivity and a Life Path 2 is especially sensitive to the needs of others. This is a good thing. My husband has a two in his numerology and sometimes knows better than me what I need. It is so lovely to have someone anticipate your needs! But the other side of this same tendency is not so nicey-nice. If a two becomes co-dependent and puts EVERYONES needs before their own this can cause issues. Not just for the Life Path 2 themselves, but for the receiver. When a Life Path 2 feels responsible for someone and tries to help (was not asked or helps too much) and gets rejected they may have feelings of resentment.

Make copies of the following pages to make notes and to calculate the numerology for any word or your name. Be sure to include your initial thoughts and feelings upon discovering this information.

1	2	3	4	5	6	7	8	9
A	B	C	D	E	F	G	H	I
J	K	L	M	N	O	P	Q	R
S	T	U	V	W	X	Y	Z	

ATTRIBUTES OF THE NUMBER

One

1	2	3	4	5	6	7	8	9
A	B	C	D	E	F	G	H	I
J	K	L	M	N	O	P	Q	R
S	T	U	V	W	X	Y	Z	

1   *represents the letters A, J and S*

Authority

Beginning

Benevolence

Creativity

Leadership

ATTRIBUTES OF THE NUMBER

One

1	2	3	4	5	6	7	8	9
A	B	C	D	E	F	G	H	I
J	K	L	M	N	O	P	Q	R
S	T	U	V	W	X	Y	Z	

1 *represents the letters A, J and S*

New

Physical body

Positive

Protection

Resources

ATTRIBUTES OF THE NUMBER

Two

1	2	3	4	5	6	7	8	9
A	B	C	D	E	F	G	H	I
J	K	L	M	N	O	P	Q	R
S	T	U	V	W	X	Y	Z	

2 *represents the letters B, K and T*

Balance

Caring

Cheerful

Conception

Dreams

ATTRIBUTES OF THE NUMBER

Two

1	2	3	4	5	6	7	8	9
A	B	C	D	E	F	G	H	I
J	K	L	M	N	O	P	Q	R
S	T	U	V	W	X	Y	Z	

2 *represents the letters B, K and T*

Emotions

Feelings

Moon

Romantic

Sensitive

ATTRIBUTES OF THE NUMBER
Three

1	2	3	4	5	6	7	8	9
A	B	C	D	E	F	G	H	I
J	K	L	M	N	O	P	Q	R
S	T	U	V	W	X	Y	Z	

3 *represented by the letters C, L, and U*

Adaptable

Charming

Creative

Idealistic

Initiative

ATTRIBUTES OF THE NUMBER

Three

1	2	3	4	5	6	7	8	9
A	B	C	D	E	F	G	H	I
J	K	L	M	N	O	P	Q	R
S	T	U	V	W	X	Y	Z	

3 *represented by the letters C, L, U*

Popular

Service

Social

Versatile

Write

ATTRIBUTES OF THE NUMBER

Four

1	2	3	4	5	6	7	8	9
A	B	C	D	E	F	G	H	I
J	K	L	M	N	O	P	Q	R
S	T	U	V	W	X	Y	Z	

4 *represents the letters D, M and V*

Building

Foundations

Hardworking

Logical

Loyal

ATTRIBUTES OF THE NUMBER

Four

1	2	3	4	5	6	7	8	9
A	B	C	D	E	F	G	H	I
J	K	L	M	N	O	P	Q	R
S	T	U	V	W	X	Y	Z	

4 *represents the letters D, M and V*

Material

Reliability

Solid

Step-by-Step

Thoughtful

ATTRIBUTES OF THE NUMBER

Five

1	2	3	4	5	6	7	8	9
A	B	C	D	E	F	G	H	I
J	K	L	M	N	O	P	Q	R
S	T	U	V	W	X	Y	Z	

5 *represents the letters E, N and W*

Change

Discipline

Education

Expansion

Freedom

ATTRIBUTES OF THE NUMBER
Five

1	2	3	4	5	6	7	8	9
A	B	C	D	E	F	G	H	I
J	K	L	M	N	O	P	Q	R
S	T	U	V	W	X	Y	Z	

5 *represents the letters E, N and W*

Intellect

Movement

Regeneration

Tolerance

Travel

ATTRIBUTES OF THE NUMBER

Six

1	2	3	4	5	6	7	8	9
A	B	C	D	E	F	G	H	I
J	K	L	M	N	O	P	Q	R
S	T	U	V	W	X	Y	Z	

6 *represents the letters F, O and X*

Beauty

Business

Discriminatory

Domestic

Effective

ATTRIBUTES OF THE NUMBER

Six

1	2	3	4	5	6	7	8	9
A	B	C	D	E	F	G	H	I
J	K	L	M	N	O	P	Q	R
S	T	U	V	W	X	Y	Z	

6   *represents the letters F, O and X*

Fantasy

Harmony

Intuition

Luxury

Unconditional Love

ATTRIBUTES OF THE NUMBER

Seven

1	2	3	4	5	6	7	8	9
A	B	C	D	E	F	G	H	I
J	K	L	M	N	O	P	Q	R
S	T	U	V	W	X	Y	Z	

7 *represents the letters G, P and Y*

Bridge

Communications

Faith

Knowledge

Limits

ATTRIBUTES OF THE NUMBER

Seven

1	2	3	4	5	6	7	8	9
A	B	C	D	E	F	G	H	I
J	K	L	M	N	O	P	Q	R
S	T	U	V	W	X	Y	Z	

7 *represents the letters G, P and Y*

Mystic

Poetic

Spiritual

Truth

Wisdom

ATTRIBUTES OF THE NUMBER

Eight

1	2	3	4	5	6	7	8	9
A	B	C	D	E	F	G	H	I
J	K	L	M	N	O	P	Q	R
S	T	U	V	W	X	Y	Z	

8   represents the letters H, Q and Z

Abundance

Ambitious

Finance

Justice

Organized

ATTRIBUTES OF THE NUMBER

Eight

1	2	3	4	5	6	7	8	9
A	B	C	D	E	F	G	H	I
J	K	L	M	N	O	P	Q	R
S	T	U	V	W	X	Y	Z	

8   *represents the letters H, Q and Z*

Persistence

Power

Self sufficient

Subconscious

Transformational

ATTRIBUTES OF THE NUMBER

Nine

1	2	3	4	5	6	7	8	9
A	B	C	D	E	F	G	H	I
J	K	L	M	N	O	P	Q	R
S	T	U	V	W	X	Y	Z	

9   *represents letters I and R*

Compassionate

Completion

Divine Love

Endings

Fun

ATTRIBUTES OF THE NUMBER

Nine

1	2	3	4	5	6	7	8	9
A	B	C	D	E	F	G	H	I
J	K	L	M	N	O	P	Q	R
S	T	U	V	W	X	Y	Z	

9   *represents letters I and R*

Future

Humanitarian

Inspirational

Originality

Talent

It does take time and effort to have a deep understanding of your true self no matter which method you chose. For me, it has spanned five years with numerology and continues. You can do the majority of the work on your own and/or have in-depth readings done by a Numerologist. Each time you review your numerology, a little more of yourself will be revealed. This is why numerology is my go to. While numerology can get complicated like dream interpretation, it can also be simplistic. This is where I come in. The idea of this book is to present it in an easy to follow format. If you can add eight single digit numbers, you can do your own numerology. I have broken down its meaning and applied it for you.

Read on so you can see what fits into your life and apply it. Use your mind to absorb the words and your heart to decide what is best for you.

CHAPTER 2

How Numbers Can
Promote Your Fitness

"If you knew your potential to feel good, you would ask
no one to be different so that you can feel good."
ESTER HICKS

We are not talking Cross Fit or Tri-athlete here or six pack abs. We are talking about incorporating fitness into your life with ease and grace. These approaches are not the run of the mill, they are tried and true methods to help you get the desired level of fitness you crave. If you do want rock hard abs, you can find them here. If you want to get off the couch, you can find that here too.

The most important thing you need to understand is the moment you intend on doing something, those thoughts put things into motion. It is the negative thoughts which undo the effort. If you are going to be successful, you need to decide you will be successful. Part of your daily "workout" will be checking your thoughts. It is very important. This cannot be stressed enough. Consider a negative thought as Superman would consider kryptonite. Negative thoughts are kryptonite. Negative statements about your progress is kryptonite on crack. You must work to overcome those negative thoughts, the same as you work your muscles. Negative thought is any thought which does not serve your greatest and highest good. Another definition of a negative thought, is any statement you do not want to be true or is self- limiting. For example, if you hear yourself say, "I am fat." Do you want this to be true? Stop saying it if you do not want it to be your truth.

It is helpful to understand how your brain works when we talk about negative thoughts. Did you ever consider where thoughts come from? Do they appear out of nowhere? Well, we do not really need to know where your thoughts come from to understand we can control them. The makings of a TV are very complex, most of us do not know *how* it works, but it is very easy to turn off. When a negative thought enters your brain, say "control alt delete", "this is not truth", or "this is not *my* truth." Immediately replace with a positive thought. Another way to reprogram your brain is by adding positive affirmations. You can get crazy with these and most often the craziest of them works the best. "I have a rock hard body." "I have the best booty on the block." And so on. Try to make your positive affirmations personal, either making yourself laugh or cry (joyful tears) so a physical or emotional reaction happens when you make the statement. This reaction is called desire and it feels really good.

Yet another approach is to tape record some positive thoughts for yourself for those days you are not in the mood or cannot think of anything positive. Allow quiet space in between your statements or story if you prefer, so you can add positive thoughts in between. When I say "story", I mean you can elaborate on your statements of affirmation. Like "My body is so sexy, the bus boy dropped his tray when he was looking at me." "I am healthy, so much so my Doctor fired me because I no longer require appointments." "I have saved so much money on health care, I am taking myself on a vacation."

When you first start, you may not catch yourself every time you have a negative thought, this is okay. You are undoing several years of bad habits. If you are the type of person who does not say negative things to yourself, this is great. Whether you use negative statements or not, an assessment of your situation can be deemed by looking at your 'to do' lists and ask yourself why it is not completed. This lack of follow through on things you want to accomplish is a clue. Where you have resistance in your life (things you are not completing) there is negativity surrounding it.

This negativity can be dispelled. Now that you have a positive platform to start off your new approach to health and wellness, here is your Health and Wellness Numerology to help you with your fitness plan.

To calculate your Health and Wellness Path add all the digits of your birth date until you get a single digit. Make copies of these pages if this is not your book or if you would like to calculate more than five birth dates.

Example:

$$August\ 4,\ 1969$$
$$8 + 4 + 1 + 9 + 6 + 9 = 37$$
$$3 + 7 = 10$$
$$1 + 0 = 1$$
$$(Month) + (Day) + (Year) = Life\ Path$$

(___ + ___) + (___ + ___) + (__ + __ + __ + __) = _____
　Day　　　　　Month　　　　　　Year

_____ + _____ = ___

Life Path/Health and Wellness Path

Be sure to double check your math.

HEALTH AND WELLNESS PATH WORKSHEET

$$(\underline{\quad} + \underline{\quad}) + (\underline{\quad} + \underline{\quad}) + (\underline{\quad} + \underline{\quad} + \underline{\quad} + \underline{\quad}) = \underline{\qquad}$$
Day   Month   Year

$$\underline{\qquad} + \underline{\qquad} = \underline{\quad}$$

Health and Wellness Path

$$(\underline{\quad} + \underline{\quad}) + (\underline{\quad} + \underline{\quad}) + (\underline{\quad} + \underline{\quad} + \underline{\quad} + \underline{\quad}) = \underline{\qquad}$$
Day   Month   Year

$$\underline{\qquad} + \underline{\qquad} = \underline{\quad}$$

Health and Wellness Path

HEALTH AND WELLNESS PATH WORKSHEET

(__ + __) + (__ + __) + (__ + __ + __ + __) = _____
     Day   Month   Year

_____ + _____ = ___

Health and Wellness Path

(__ + __) + (__ + __) + (__ + __ + __ + __) = _____
     Day   Month   Year

_____ + _____ = ___

Health and Wellness Path

1 Health and Wellness Path

Because of your creative and expressive nature you need more than the average amount of exercise each day. Since you spend much time alone and much time in your head, chose an activity which is simple and easy to follow, dare I say "mindless"? Walking, hiking, swimming, or restorative yoga are good choices. Also, try mixing in activities you enjoyed as a child: riding a bike, roller-skating, jumping rope, cartwheels, or hula-hoop. The more playful and silly the better! Find some kids to show you how.

These ideas seem simple, but do not discount their simplicity. You will need to give your mind a break which allows for other things to come in. If your exercise choices have you counting and keeping track, it will distract you from the reason you need to exercise. In addition to the fitness aspect of exercise, your mind will get the break it needs. Your body needs to burn off some of the excess energy you have. The excess energy will be used against you if you do not burn it off. It will come at you as cravings, urges and the like. You will best be suited for an exercise you get lost in. Not because you are keeping track of it, but because you are enjoying it. Now I may lose many of you to the simplicity of your regimen, but please first try it for some time before you decide you will get bored. You will not and you will look forward to working out so long as you don't have to keep a diary of it.

Ones wanting to lose weight need to look at portion size. You will increase your exercise naturally because you like the challenge, so your focus needs to be on calories. It is best to follow a diet light on the red meats and cheeses, these are difficult for you to digest and you will think you are hungry when you are actually thirsty. (People often confuse the sensation in the stomach when digestion is taking place and needs hydration. Most think this sensation is hunger- it is actually thirst. True hunger is felt in the throat area.) A good rule of thumb for all ones is to have a variety of foods available. When you make unhealthy choices it is because a delicious healthy option is not available.

Once ones get over the hump of 7-10 weeks, a new way of eating will feel natural. As long as you can stick to the new plan. When it comes to choosing carbs, ones need to limit bread, consuming it once or twice a month. Another thing to limit is pasta. Ones will crave sweets after eating pasta so it is best not to test yourself too much in the beginning. When you get a good sense of your system running without cravings, you will have better control when cravings show up.

Ideas of exercises to mix into walking:

- 100 Quick Steps- walk as fast as you can, counting 100 steps.
- Alternating Push Offs- push off your toes, counting to 50 on each foot.
- Toe Walking- walk on your toes, work up to 100 steps.
- Thigh Driving- concentrate on using your thigh muscle all the way through your step. Do one leg at a time, working up to 100 steps.
- Walk Backwards- up hill is a great challenge, nice change up on treadmill (use hand rails!).

HEALTH AND WELLNESS
PATH JOURNAL SPACE
PATH 1

2 Health and Wellness Path

You need exercise to release muscular tension, requires attention to breath and balance. Examples: yoga, Pilates, step aerobics, sex-ooh, this is tension releasing and deep breathing! Include independent activities for yourself and above all choose what YOU like. Try uplifting movement with music, dancing, or deep breathing. Add beauty to your workout by choosing appealing colors and fabrics you wear to workout. Consider how you can beautify the surroundings. Include stretching and meditation **every day.** If the idea of meditation does not appeal to you let me give you some tidbits. First, meditation does not have to be long. Secondly, it is not necessary to try to 'clear your mind'. By putting your mind on one thing, you are doing a form of meditation. If your mind wanders, bring it back. Your mind will wander, this is not 'failure' on your part. Do not judge yourself when your mind does this. The awareness that your mind wandered is the work. Therefore, catching yourself when your mind wanders *is* what meditation is about. Here are some mediation ideas to get you started. Please try them.

Five Minute Meditation Ideas

- Dry Brushing- before showering, use a dry brush on your entire body. Your goal is to keep your mind where your brush is (on your body) and offer positive thoughts with each brush stroke.
- Forehead Down- on a desk or table, fold your arms on top of each other, placing your forehead on arms, scoot your chair back until comfortable. Breathe here until you feel complete.
- Mind In Your Body- sit or lay comfortably, starting at your head, putting your mind in each body part as you make your way down your body. Stay in each body part as long as you like or until you feel a sensation.
- I Love My Feet- before bed, massage your feet with lotion or oil. As you work, thank your feet for all they do for you.
- Love My Hands- do this any time of the day, especially if you use your hands for work. Massage them and thank them for all the tasks they attend to.

I need to repeat, the exercise you choose needs to be something you want to do. You will soon see, it is in the choosing, you fail yourself.

Let's make this clear, pretend you only get one chance to choose. Imagine you can only pick one kind of exercise, only one. Close your eyes, take a few breaths and choose. Now, what did you choose? You can also know by choosing what it is you truly desire, in itself, is a lesson for you. You will not do anyone any good if you continue to make choices based on what others think or what others want.

As a two, your only problem losing weight is when you create limits for yourself. If you only have thirty minutes to walk because your schedule is too full, you do not get the benefits of a sixty minute walk. It is best if you allow yourself more time and stop when you feel like it. "Feeling" is the key here. When you allow yourself to feel, you will soon be able to use this as your guide and be true to yourself. Honoring yourself in this way will inspire much weight loss.

When twos make food choices, consider the area in which it is consumed. It is important the environment be peaceful to fully enjoy the meal. A better connection will be made. Consider talking to your food. This might sound crazy, heck it looks crazy, but it creates a relationship. No need to talk out loud, only to pause for a moment to set an intention. Tell the food to nourish your body fully and to bring all the energy necessary. If you can create a loving relationship between your food and body, (balance) you will no longer struggle with your weight. This relationship is one of creating balance which is one of your lessons in life.

Affirmations: "My food goes into my body creating all the energy I need. I love my food and what it can do for my body."

HEALTH AND WELLNESS
PATH JOURNAL SPACE
PATH 2

3 Health and Wellness Path

Expressive movement suits you best, like Zumba or interpretive dance. Find inspiring energetic music or write your own. Choose music to mirror your current feelings and move with it. Consider teaching, leading or creating a fitness class. Your creativity and enthusiasm alone make you qualified for such an endeavor. A few places you can shine: MeetUp.com, Baby and Me fitness club, or a neighborhood park. Share the price of a babysitter with a group of friends and workout at the park.

Threes are sometimes competitive, with an internal need to show others what you can do. This is good for somethings, but not for your overall physical fitness. In general, playing a game such as golf, volleyball or bowling should not count as exercise, it will not be enough. Moving each day in the manner of your mood, will be very helpful. If you are signed up for a game, requiring you to run back and forth and it is a day you would rather dance, this outlet will not help. You need to stay in-tuned to the yearnings of your body, listen to it and do as it asks. Some days your body will only ask to be stretched, some days it will need to run a marathon. Well, not an actual marathon, but it may need to extend itself past preconceived limits, for emotional energies can be trapped and need to be pounded out. If you get the feeling "Oh I need to go for a run," do it. Wear good shoes and run as much as you can tolerate. Stretch well afterwards and take a bath or get a massage. Your body needs you to listen to it, it has much more good information for you if you do.

Once a routine of 4-5 days a week for a month has been accomplished, you can begin to limit foods. No single food (sweet, salty, savory) is usually the culprit. Most of all, threes like to eat. This is good as it creates a good relationship with food. What you need to do is consider where food comes from and what work went into producing it and getting it to you. When you understand most meals do not "grow on trees" you will have a greater respect for what is on the plate. Participating in the process of a meal fully helps you will realize, a great amount of energy went into its preparation, thus forging the respect even further.

If you want to cut down on how much you eat or change what choices are made, it is best to become more involved with the process. Learn more about food in general by reading packages. If you do not recognize a word on the ingredient list, look it up. If you make it a rule never to eat anything you do not recognize, you will never have to worry about weight. When you tire of reading packages, your food choices will be fresh fruits and veggies…beautiful.

Threes occasionally need to do a cleanse. Not the crazy "no food for days on end" type of cleanse, but a gentle one. It can be a juice cleanse or a water fast, but only for a day or two. This will help you respect food and what it does for your body. It will also give your system a much needed break. Flushing the body with pure water is good, adding a little lemon is even better. There are many great websites by doctors and nutritionist with good guidelines. Or consult with a qualified doctor to make the best choice. If you check in with your own doctor, and are advised against it, find another doctor who supports you.

HEALTH AND WELLNESS
PATH JOURNAL SPACE
PATH 3

4 Health and Wellness Path

Step-by-step and goal oriented fitness program works best for you. Sign up for a half marathon and train for it. Make it a goal to be a black belt within 2 years, etc. Also weight training, running, and biking are good choices. Does competition motivate you? Try a sport like tennis or racquetball.

Fours also like to boss people around so a fitness regimen requiring you to give some direction would be good. If you could lead a team in a vigorous exercise this would be the best for you. Being the captain of a basketball team or the leader of a marching band, (forgive the pun) are well-orchestrated examples. You need your mind counting, figuring and fixing so your body can get involved. This brain/body connection is so strong, it is best not to separate the two.

When a four needs to amp things up, get a fitness trainer. Trainers are very step-by-step, regimented and will keep you on your game. It is a good match and fours will enjoy all the counting, keeping track and follow up trainers do. Another helpful thing for you is to have a sense of what is to be accomplished. If you want to lose weight, you will enjoy the math of calories in, calories out. Here is something to get fours started:

Step 1- Check your calendar, mark the days and times you have available to exercise.

Step 2- Pick a physical activity you like.

Step 3- Look online for classes/meet up groups/clubs coinciding with the list you made.

Step 4- Go to the Organizing chapter and use it to complete your fitness schedule.

HEALTH AND WELLNESS
PATH JOURNAL SPACE
PATH 4

5 Health and Wellness Path

You will get the freedom you need when you create a disciplined approach to your fitness program. Freedom from health worries, freedom to sleep well, freedom in your diet choices, etc. Variety in fitness is very important. If you are missing work outs or do not work out at all, it is due to boredom. Something simple as walking can be changed up by going at a different time of day, different location, adding music, books on tape or comedy (free on Pandora). Do not do the same work out two days in a row. Being regimented does not mean being boring. Try fast moving aerobics class, Zumba, etcetera. You don't have to be super fit or know how to dance to enjoy this class! Note: if you are talking a lot during a class you are bored. If you enjoy talking while working out, use ear buds and microphone and talk while walking outside, not indoors, this is annoying to do around others.

Fives will also benefit from having a selection of workout equipment. It is best to have things you know how to use and you are willing to do. It is best to have equipment set up where you can see it every day. For most people the equipment will collect dust, but not for a five. You like to have different things to do at different times. This will encourage you to do more workouts, more often.

Set up a workout room. You can even do this in a section of the living room. You need not worry about it cramping your life style, feeling good is part of everyone's life style. Be prepared to loan out your equipment because others around you will want to share. This gives you an excuse to buy more interesting equipment when you get bored with what you have. If money is an issue, go to garage sales and get second hand items. Trade fitness equipment with friends, family and neighbors. Variety is the spice of life!

Fives, you will do well for yourself by picking movements you are best at physically. Like using your hands. You can bet you will enjoy some time at the gym, but in limited amounts. You can get a membership if it is affordable, but most likely attending too many of the same type of classes will make you angry. Boredom will be avoided if you keep changing your workouts. This is a mandatory thing. You must not have the same work out two days in a row- ever! No matter how much you liked it.

When Fives need to lose weight it is most likely due to making unhealthy food choices in a big way. You like to have many options. The world is full of food options so you pick all of them. When it comes to food you really need to limit choices per meal. A little of this, a little of that and before you know it you have two meals on your plate. What you need to do is: one protein, one carb, two or three veggie/fruit. When observing serving size and having a different meal each time, fives will find success in weight loss. It is best to limit the foods which give you a heavy feeling or weighs you down. To become more aware of this, reduce the choices on your plate. You will know it was the pork and not the chicken, the cheese not potatoes. You can tune into your body and eventually only eat what is needed.

HEALTH AND WELLNESS
PATH JOURNAL SPACE
PATH 5

6 Health and Wellness Path

Pick any physical activity you *think* you are not very good at and do it anyway. Guess what, it will be perfect because it is good for you. Notice how you **feel** while you exercise. Picture running like Phoebe in the "Friends" episode, an anything goes kind of attitude. Try Tai Chi or something similar so you can slow down and enjoy the process. Like to golf? Do not take a cart, do not keep score, and while you are walking between holes, notice the surroundings.

Other type of activities requiring skills are also good. You like to learn new things and after you get over the initial "I can't do this" you will be great at it. You are best suited for activities requiring you to pay closer attention. Dance with someone, as opposed to by yourself. Play doubles tennis instead of one on one. When you pay attention to the others it will take focus off yourself. If you can take a gymnastics class, (Yes there is gymnastics for adults with no prior experience! It is super fun too!) you will be concentrating on the instruction, keeping your balance and so forth, so time will go by very fast and you will be working hard.

Sixes may not do so well on self-directed activities as your mind tends to wander and you will think of other things to do. Best bet is to schedule and pay for a work out. You will be sure not to miss it, or be late *and* you will want to get your money's worth. If money is an issue, plan and schedule workouts with friends. Accountability is key for you.

A six trying to lose weight needs emotional support while making those changes. The support does not have to be a clinical or cost hundreds per hour, but you will need to have help with all the emotions coming out of you along the process. A group like Weight Watchers (Don't eat the food!), Overeaters Anonymous, etc. A place where you feel safe, supported, not judged and offered unconditional love. This is so you can express your feelings, which is most likely why you are making unhealthy choices. Also, when your body starts to detox and you have given it the green light to release what does not serve you, stuff might start flying out like gang busters. Being aware of this will help, you are not losing your mind. Yes, it feels like it. Have support when it does, which will help even more with your wellness goals.

HEALTH AND WELLNESS
PATH JOURNAL SPACE
PATH 6

7 Health and Wellness Path

Do as many outdoor activities as possible. Mix in something you enjoy requiring your attention, concentration, counting or that builds upon proceeding classes. Try dancing, Gymnastics, Kickboxing, or Martial arts.

Sevens will do well to keep up with the popular trend. You like to know what is going on and will be able to keep up with whatever the new "dance craze" is. The ability to tell everyone how the new fitness gadget works, will help you with your own fitness goals. Occasionally getting on friends nerves with your enthusiasm is bound to happen, do not worry about it. You encourage others to get fit.

What sevens like best is to be able to get a workout done fast. You have much to do and do not like to lollygag at anything. A quick powerful workout is what is needed. The ideal workout is one requiring lifting body parts repeatedly. It is in your best interest to make a plan and stick to it. Sevens also do best when you make a commitment. A membership will be good motivation and you can enjoy all the new equipment and classes. If you have a seven in your life and want to get in shape, ask them to help you. A seven will become the cheerleader you need to keep you motivated. Sevens also enjoy the company and sharing all their fitness wisdom.

When a seven has completely given up on a workout routine it is most likely due to health issues. If you do not feel well, you will not want to exercise. This can be detrimental to a seven, as the need to move and breath is very important. It is best for a seven to figure out what is causing the health issue, most likely something to do with back, breathing, or lungs. Sevens carry the weight of the world and this causes much discomfort. Seeking medical/healing attention (not drugs) for the pain will be beneficial to start. As you feel better, slip in exercise here and there until you are fully recovered. If you are a seven, let the pain be a lesson, learn from it and get yourself into shape. You have a lot of work to do.

HEALTH AND WELLNESS
PATH JOURNAL SPACE
PATH 7

8 Health and Wellness Path

Tapping into your inner abundance and power is the key to your fitness routine. Be a workout buddy, inspire and encourage others to exercise. Sharing in this area will certainly motivate yourself and others to meet fitness goals. Can you share your abundance with others by offering a free class or volunteer to teach? Good choices are: Martial arts, weight lifting, kickboxing, and tennis.

As an eight, you can out do most people, you are built this way. Occasionally this propensity to drive yourself causes a problem, making you over-do it. Sometimes overdoing to the point you do not want to do it again for a long while. You become frustrated with the lack of energy, because you do not understanding there is not an endless supply of it. When you get a routine, you will see you have more energy for the occasional power day. As an eight, you make good marathon runners if you pace yourself in the days leading up to the race. If you try to do too much leading up to it, you will wear yourself out. If an eight can get past the need to outperform everyone every time, a relaxed fitness routine will become part of life. Competition has its place, but eights need to be aware of being overly competitive all the time. When you work out with a partner you do not need to win at everything. You will lose out on the process of getting fit if you make it a competition.

As an eight, you will have a good time doing anything you chose and you are best at things not calling for much thought. So much thinking energy being used all day, when it comes time to be physical it is best to do something less thinking. When the routine gets too routine, switch it up. Taking on sports with the seasons is good. Skiing in the winter, running in the Spring and Summer. Keep a pattern so you can get right back into what you had done before.

HEALTH AND WELLNESS
PATH JOURNAL SPACE
PATH 8

9 Health and Wellness Path

Gee, you are good at so many things. What to choose, what to choose? You lead others without trying, imagine what you can do if you made a conscious attempt at it? Place your physical efforts into activities like Habitat for Humanity, Big Brothers Big Sisters, coaching youth sports or any outdoor activity: hunting, fishing or weekend camping trips.

You have so much self-leadership it is difficult to give you advice on the subject of yourself. You would do best to make an example of your workout regimen for others, thus the suggestion for Big Brother/ Big Sister program. You can arrive at a place where the thought of working out is less desirable. The main motivation will be vanity, you like to stay looking good. Whatever your motivation, it is best to follow it. You can get into all sorts of trouble if energy is not use for the greatest and highest good. You can be prone to addictions if you are not aware of this. Time alone to process things and plenty of quiet time is important. Vary your exercise to fit your mood or energy level. Also you will find it most beneficial to do Tai Chi and the like. You have so many emotions going through you all the time, like the sensitivity of the twos, but with more depth. You need to burn some of it off. At other times, an easy walk all alone will be enough. Many nines can be found sitting still, you love to sit. You can sit for hours. Most nines do not need to be told to meditate, often it is natural to quietly contemplate or see what comes up. Nines can be one of the calmest of the numbers, but remember lots can be going on underneath the surface. Picture an iceberg.

HEALTH AND WELLNESS
PATH JOURNAL SPACE
PATH 9

Talk to your doctor before starting any new fitness program. Consult professional trainers when necessary.

Free work out ideas:

- Rent work out videos from library- get several at a time.
- Free exercise aps or for little cost.
- YouTube videos
- Instagram
- Pinterest

If you have kids:

- Make an obstacle course with chalk: skip, hop scotch, jumping jacks, etc.
- Jump rope; Chinese jump rope (draw two lines on sidewalk) or double dutch
- T-ball (Place a foam ball on an orange safety cone for hitting success.)
- Play catch- I have yet to meet a kid that refuses a game of catch. Use balled up socks, bean bags, Koosh ball, water balloon, small stuffed animal, or tennis ball
- Frisbee
- Basketball game using the laundry basket with above mentioned items.
- Get activity book from the library and let the kids pick.

My thoughts on Yoga

There was a time not long ago when I would have rather put a sharp object in my eye than do yoga. Now, I would be tempted to use the same sharp object on anyone who would prevent me from doing yoga. I have actually heard people say; "I can't do yoga because I am not flexible." Your lack of flexibility is the REASON to take yoga. You will continue the imbalance and create crazy misalignments in your body. It is too bad many get the impression yoga aficionados are all flexible- this is not true. I have had teachers point out, "Tricia you are so flexible in your back and legs, but your hips are so tight." Yes, precisely why I take yoga, for my hips!

Go to each yoga class with the attitude of 'what will I learn about myself today?' A good yoga teacher can help you get the most of it. If your teacher is not making adjustments on you each class- ask to have adjustments made. If a class your attending is not making adjustments on your postures either verbally or physically, FIND ANOTHER TEACHER! I have seen veteran yoga instructors get adjustments from other instructors- yes! Do I think the instructors receiving the adjustments lack knowledge? Heck no, and it explains yoga as a process, a life time long process, and you may never get every position *perfect*. This is okay because the feeling you get after a restorative yoga class is marvelous- similar to the yummy glow you have after a massage.

Just one more thing on yoga being a process. When I first started virasana or hero pose, I needed two blocks stacked under me and sometimes towels behind my knees. In three years of a regular practice (two classes a week) I can now sit for a short time on one block. Some might say this is slow progress, for me it is a small miracle.

CHAPTER **3**

How to Organize Yourself

"You don't go shopping with a list of things you don't want."
KENNETH LADFORD

Organizing Your New Fitness Goals

In this step of the process you will be making tools to help you organize your new fitness goals. You can consider these tools as you would glue for a puzzle. You have all the pieces, you have put them together now you need to make them stick so your hard work does not fall apart.

The first tool you will make is organizing oracle cards. This will be an exciting endeavor because the energy of your intent (Your goals are your intent!) will be added to the cards as you create them. The process of making your own cards will deepen your connection to them. They will be your 'calling card' to the Universe, making it clear what you desire. This is important because your **intent** to create health with your fitness program strengthens your resolve. This energy will be all over the cards you make. Exciting!

Decorate the backside of your cards or leave them blank, it is up to you. Adding a creative flair will further deepen the connection to their meaning and energy. Also, it is just plain old fun to get crafty. The front side of the card will be data you fill in. This data will be a combination of your current level of fitness, your fitness goals and your Health and Wellness Path information. The cards will be divided into three sections: frequency, duration and activity.

Follow these steps to create your own organizing oracle cards. The following steps will show you how to use them to make a fitness schedule.

Chose which method you would like to use to make your cards:

o   Make your own with index cards
o   Photo copy the templates from the end of this chapter
o   Download from www.TriciasEnergyGarden.com

What you will need to make your own cards:

✓   30 or more Index cards, any size, 3 different colors or add color to plain white
✓   Fun markers, pencils or ink pens

Back of cards: (Optional) Use the following ideas to decorate the backside of your oracle cards:

o   Print out your numerology art at www.TriciasEnergyGarden.com
o   Cut and glue on inspiring photos from magazines
o   Use your makers, pencils and pens to add personal art
o   Tech savvy and have a printer? Design them online, in Publisher or as a Word document

You will make three cards for each section, a total of six cards. Keep all of the unused supplies and Index cards. You will add cards as you move forward in the program or as you discover fun new things to add to your workout regime.

Based your current level of workouts, decide which category fits you best. Underestimating how much you workout is better, this leaves room for improvement.

FITNESS CATAGORY

Beginner	Intermediate	Proficient
Zero- 1	3-4	4-7
workouts per week	workouts per week	workouts per week
occasionally exercises	semi- regular workouts	rarely misses a workout

What is your current Fitness Category?

How do you feel about your current level of fitness?

What is your ultimate goal?

Explore your feelings here:

Below is a frequency, duration and activity chart. Thus the need for having 3 different colors of cards to represent, "frequency", "duration" and "activity". This is the structure we will use to build your program. You will make a minimum of 3 cards in each section. (Side note: This is a remake of the meditation program I created for myself. It is how I added meditation to my life. My meditation practice started out at only two times a month. That was four years ago, I really enjoyed the process and have progressed to doing two meditations a day sometimes. I no longer require the cards as a prompt!)

FREQUENCY

Beginner	Intermediate	Proficient
3 x's a month	2x's a week	6x's a week
5 x's a month	3x's a week	7x's a week
7 x's a month	4 x's a week	2 works outs daily

What is your current Frequency?

How do you feel about your current level of frequency?

What is your ultimate goal?

Explore your feelings here:

DURATION

Beginner	Intermediate	Proficient
10 minutes	30 minutes	60 minutes
15 minutes	40 minutes	70 minutes
20 minutes	50 minutes	*80 minutes

*This is a professional or training athlete. Days off to recover will be necessary but your days 'off' will be leisurely walks, restorative Yoga, Tai Chi, or stretching.

In your Duration section, one card will be your current amount of time you usually spend working out, the second card will increase 5 minutes, the third card will increase by 10 minutes.

What is your current level of duration?

How do you feel about your current level of fitness?

What is your ultimate goal?

Explore your feelings here:

ACTIVITY

Beginner	Intermediate	Proficient
Zero- 1	3-4	4-7
workouts per week	workouts per week	workouts per week
occasionally exercises	semi- regular	rarely misses a
	workouts	workout

Refer to your Health and Wellness Path number. Please make copies of the Journal page provided and make your notes.

HEALTH AND WELLNESS
PATH ACTIVITY LIST:

Feel free to make as many Activity cards as you would like at this time but only include three cards when you are ready to create your fitness schedule. The majority of the Activity cards you make need to be activities you enjoy. Several of the cards need to be something that you have never done. One or two of the cards need to be activities you feel resistance to or have not considered. Trust any card you pull is meant to be added to your workouts, it is something that will serve your greatest and highest good.

Creating Your Fitness Schedule

After you have made all of your cards you are ready to begin the next step.

Chose one card, at random from each section. You will then have one card from Frequency, one card from Duration and one card from Activity. You now have the structure you need to create your fitness schedule. Trust that the cards you pulled at random is the best scenario for you.

Example:

> Health and Wellness Path 8 at the Beginner Level who is currently working out 1 day a week for 10 minutes would make the following cards:
>
> ❖ **Frequency Cards:**
> - 4 times a month (current level of frequency)
> - 5 times a month
> - 6 times a month
>
> ❖ **Duration Cards:**
> - 10 minutes (current level)
> - 15 minutes
> - 20 minutes
>
> ❖ **Activity Cards:**
> - Walking (winter activity)
> - Swimming (summer activity)

Added cards:

- Workout with partner
- Dancing (favorite activity)
- Stretching

The cards picked at random for this Health and Wellness Path 8 example are:

Frequency- 6 times a month
Duration- 15 minutes
Activity- Walking

The fitness schedule for this 8 Path is to walk 15 minutes 1-2 times per week. Alternating one time a week with two times a week would make 6 workouts in one month. If you reached your goal for the month use your cards to make a new schedule for the next month. If you fell short on your goal this month, review your notes, make changes if needed and repeat the goal of 6 times a month until it has become an easy habit. Make a copy of the following blank schedule before completing your next step.

	Sunday	Monday	Tues.	Wed.	Thurs.	Friday	Sat.
Current Schedule							
Added Schedule							

How to Work with Your Oracle Cards

When you first start with your cards remember you only need to set an intention. There is no magic here, it is pure intention. The energy we spoke of before that is in the numbers, it is in you and around you. The same energy that attracts beautiful friends to you, is the same energy that will attract the correct cards to you. The reason it seems like a 'woo woo' thing is because the ability has been programed out of you. You do have this ability, to know what you need to take care of yourself. It is in every human being. Trust that it is in you.

Also consider you are simply writing a list of things that are good for you and using the process of elimination to create your new schedule. It is that simple. The oracle cards will be your list and you will 'mark them off' as you go along. They are in the form of cards to block out any outside influences. Another way I like to think about it, is you are your own boss. You wrote your list and now you are deciding what needs to be done on your list, similar to what your boss does for you at work.

When you are ready to start, select the number of cards that seems right to you. I will give you guidelines but if you "hear" the number three pop into your head, only do 3 cards at a time. If you had accidently dropped all of your cards and five were face up, use five cards. The important part is that you do not feel overwhelmed or confused.

Think of this as synchronicity at its finest. Yes, we are directing the outcome a little bit but it is not less synchronistic. I must stress, you cannot do this wrong. My first card reading I gave for someone else had taken place the same day I purchased my first deck. (Synchronicity had struck while on my lunch hour and a deck found me!) I had been in possession of my very first tarot deck for only 45 minutes. While I was in the act of preserving the cards secrecy, a coworker asked for a reading. My mind was shouting 'no' as she asked me. Having only done four Reiki healings up until that point, with no intent in adding Reiki to my resume, I sure was not ready to add tarot card readings too!

The self-doubt was squelched long enough for a reading to occur. I also could not explain the resounding "Yes!" that bolted from my face instead of the "No." As I started the reading, my mind was hearing two voices, "You cannot do this." "Shuffle the cards." "You are an idiot, what if someone finds out?" "Use the signal you get in your ears to pick cards." "You are nuts, don't you dare tell her how you picked the cards!" Fumbling and stumbling over my words like a toddler walking for the first time, feeling so off balance, yet moving forward anyway. The torture of two threads of thoughts reeling through my head, trying to choose which ones sounded *less* nuts. Then, like magic the reading came, much needed answers and reassures came, then tears of relief came. It is not magic. It is the Law of Attraction. Please use it to your advantage!

How do you feel about The Law of Attraction and tarot/oracle cards?

FREQUENCY

DURATION

ACTIVITY

CHAPTER 4

How to use Personal Year and Personal Day to amp up your resolve

"Lead with Your Truth."
CHALENE JOHNSON

Personal Year

You just learned your date of birth sheds light on what type of exercise is most appealing. Your Life Path Number can give you more information besides your life purpose. Isn't it exciting to know this *and* have those energies working for you? Your date of birth produces an energy within you and it does not stop at your Life Path Number.

Astrologers explain the influence of the planets specific to each astrology sign as well as the influence relative in all signs. The sun in Aries is specific to Aries. A full moon is broad and influences all astrological signs. The influence of the full moon is felt differently by each sign. Like astrology, numerology can be applied in a broader sense, as well. You do not need to study or memorize anything as the astrologers do, just understand numbers create an energy that in turn influences you.

In this chapter we are going to examine your Personal Year Number and Personal Day Number. Both are a single digit number (1-9) added the same way as your Health and Wellness Path Number. These numbers provide you with an 'umbrella' or an additional boost of energy to tap into. The Personal Year Number is the vibe expanding over a 12 month period. Please make copies of the calculation worksheet and the Journal pages that follow so you can make notes.

To calculate this number, add your month and day of birth with the current year until you have a single digit.

Example: August 4 + Current year

$$\text{August 4, 1969}$$
$$8 + 4 + 2 + 0 + 1 + 6 = 21$$
$$2 + 1 = 3$$
$$\text{(Month) + (Day) + (Current Year) = (Personal Year Number)}$$

(___ +___) + (___+___) + (__ + __ + __ + __) = _____
Day   Month   Current Year

_____ + _____ = ___

Personal Year Number

PERSONAL YEAR NUMBER WORKSHEET:

(__ + __) + (__ + __) + (__ + __ + __ + __) = _____
Day   Month   Current Year

_____ + _____ = ____

Personal Year Number

_____

(__ + __) + (__ + __) + (__ + __ + __ + __) = _____
Day   Month   Current Year

_____ + _____ = ____

Personal Year Number

_____

(__ + __) + (__ + __) + (__ + __ + __ + __) = _____
Day   Month   Current Year

_____ + _____ = ____

Personal Year Number

PERSONAL YEAR NUMBER WORKSHEET:

(__ + __) + (__ + __) + (__ + __ + __ + __) = _____
  Day   Month   Current Year

_____ + _____ = ____

                     Personal Year Number

(__ + __) + (__ + __) + (__ + __ + __ + __) = _____
  Day   Month   Current Year

_____ + _____ = ____

                     Personal Year Number

(__ + __) + (__ + __) + (__ + __ + __ + __) = _____
  Day   Month   Current Year

_____ + _____ = ____

                     Personal Year Number

PERSONAL YEAR NUMBER WORKSHEET:

(__ + __) + (__ + __) + (__ + __ + __ + __) = _____
   Day   Month   Current Year

_____ + _____ = ___

Personal Year Number

_____

(__ + __) + (__ + __) + (__ + __ + __ + __) = _____
   Day   Month   Current Year

_____ + _____ = ___

Personal Year Number

_____

(__ + __) + (__ + __) + (__ + __ + __ + __) = _____
   Day   Month   Current Year

_____ + _____ = ___

Personal Year Number

I am in a 3 Personal Year. Three energy is CREATIVE and E X P R E S S I V E. This sounds good, right? Well, for the most part it is, except when you do not understand the force it creates inside of you. Like a firehose with no off switch, you need to learn how to sense it and deal with it. Resisting the urge to turn it off, get angry, or feel frustrated is imperative. The creative energy produces blinding insight and an influx of ideas. This is why it is important to honor it. As I write this, I wonder how to support you when you become aware of its power. The power can knock you for a loop if you let it. Your emotions are a good indicator for you. For myself, if I embrace all the oomph it brings me by channeling it, appreciating it and using it to my best advantage, it won't knock me down. Currently, in my 3 year, during a 3 month, when I have a 3 day, all bets are off! Meaning my attention to this multiple of 3 is top priority. Incorporating tougher workouts for an outlet helps. Getting outside and having adequate quiet and rest time is very important. It would also be smart to review the Fitness Chapter for Path 3 to get workout ideas that are expressive.

Here are the guidelines for your Personal Year Numbers. Use the energy of the year you are in as a focus. Allow it to direct your fitness goals for the year. As a bonus, use it to predict what the following years hold.

PERSONAL YEAR 1
Add new things to your fitness routine.

PERSONAL YEAR 2
Include others on a more regular basis.

PERSONAL YEAR 3
Incorporate expressive exercise options.

PERSONAL YEAR 4
Add a step-by-step fitness regimen.

PERSONAL YEAR 5
Change your focus and improve physical flexibility.

PERSONAL YEAR 6
Evaluate current regimen, see where it is out of balance.

PERSONAL YEAR 7
Learn something new about fitness or how it relates to your health.

PERSONAL YEAR 8
Set goals, abundance and power is the
theme, use it to your advantage.

PERSONAL YEAR 9
Use some of your extra energy to help those in need.

My plan: add more expressive and tougher workouts this year (Personal Year 3), add a building type class next year (Personal Year 4) and look for more ways to add flexibility to my workouts in two years (Personal Year 5).

Take a few moments to figure out your plan for this year and for the next two years before moving onto the next section. Make a copy of the Personal Year Number Journal page to make notes.

PERSONAL YEAR NUMBER JOURNALING:
PERSONAL YEAR 1
I will add these new things to my fitness routine:

PERSONAL YEAR NUMBER JOURNALING:
PERSONAL YEAR 2

This is how I will include others on a more regular basis:

PERSONAL YEAR NUMBER JOURNALING:
PERSONAL YEAR 3
I will incorporate these expressive exercises:

PERSONAL YEAR NUMBER JOURNALING:
PERSONAL YEAR 4
I will add this step-by-step fitness regimen:

PERSONAL YEAR NUMBER JOURNALING:
PERSONAL YEAR 5
I will make changes and improve my physical flexibility by:

PERSONAL YEAR NUMBER JOURNALING:
PERSONAL YEAR 6

After evaluate my current regimen, I see where it is out of balance:

PERSONAL YEAR NUMBER JOURNALING:
PERSONAL YEAR 7
I will learn something new about fitness
or how it relates to my health.
Here are some ideas:

PERSONAL YEAR NUMBER JOURNALING:
PERSONAL YEAR 8
With abundance and power as my theme, I set the following goals:

PERSONAL YEAR NUMBER JOURNALING:
PERSONAL YEAR 9
Here are ways I can use my energy to help those in need:

Personal Day Number

As the Personal Year adds a vibe to the current year, the Personal Day Number adds a vibe to each individual day on the calendar. Take for instance a Personal Day Number 5. Five carries with it freedom and discipline. Think about the opposite meaning of discipline. A conscious effort is made on my part, to describe each number positively so you can see them as attributes. But stop for a moment and think about the opposite meaning of the word discipline. Yikes! Words like disorder, confusion, unruliness, and bedlam. Oh my! These will not support a good habit. This five energy has the potential to add resistance to working out because it contains both sides of discipline. If there is a strong exercise routine in place less resistance will be felt. Use this information to review your workout journal. Does it reveal a pattern of missed workouts, could this be the energy of the five? The days when workouts were most enjoyed, what was the Personal Day Number? Discovering and planning around these tendencies would help immensely.

To calculate, add your Personal Year Number (from above) to the current month and day to get your Personal Day Number. (Month) + (Day) + (Current Year) = (Personal Year Number)

Continuing with our example above:

August 4 birthday in 2016, which is in a 3 Year.
Let us use the calendar day of March 6.
3 (Personal Year) + 3 (Month) + 6 (Day of the Month) = 12, 1+2= 3

_____ (Personal Year) + _____ (Month)
+ _____ (Day of the Month)
= _____

_____ + _____ = _____

In our example, the creative energy will be flowing hard on March 6, I better have a very expressive or hard workout session. No leisurely walk on a Personal Day 3. Go for a swim, lift weights or play tennis! I will also review Health and Wellness Path 3 for some ideas to channel this extra expressive energy.

Here are the Personal Day Numbers related to your fitness:

PERSONAL DAY 1
Solo workouts on these days.

PERSONAL DAY 2
Best spent with a partner.

PERSONAL DAY 3
Without a physically challenging workout this day could be wacky.

PERSONAL DAY 4
Get some time in the gym.

PERSONAL DAY 5
S t r e t c h i n g is most beneficial.

PERSONAL DAY 6
What exercise would you LOVE to do?

PERSONAL DAY 7
Learn something new today.
Can you do 5 push-ups? 100 crunches?

PERSONAL DAY 8
Get out of bed a little early, add the extra time to your workout.

PERSONAL DAY 9
Think outside yourself, can your fitness support humanity?

PERSONAL DAY NUMBER JOURNALING:
PERSONAL DAY 1
Solo workouts ideas:

PERSONAL DAY NUMBER JOURNALING:
PERSONAL DAY 2
Partner ideas:

PERSONAL DAY NUMBER JOURNALING:
PERSONAL DAY 3
Physically challenging workout ideas:

PERSONAL DAY NUMBER JOURNALING:
PERSONAL DAY 4
What gym activity today?

PERSONAL DAY NUMBER JOURNALING:
PERSONAL DAY 5
S t r e t c h i n g ideas:

PERSONAL DAY NUMBER JOURNALING:
PERSONAL DAY 6
What exercise would I love today?

PERSONAL DAY NUMBER JOURNALING:
PERSONAL DAY 7
How many push-ups can I do? How many crunches?

PERSONAL DAY NUMBER JOURNALING:
PERSONAL DAY 8
What time will I wake to get in a workout before breakfast?

PERSONAL DAY NUMBER JOURNALING:
PERSONAL DAY 9
Can my fitness support humanity?

Here are a few more examples:

DOB July 19, 1993
7 +1 + 9 + 2 + 0 + 1 + 6 = 26 2+6= 8
Example: Personal Year 8

In this example, 2016, being a Personal Year 8, it is the year for setting new fitness goals. No status quo, increasing workout time and adding power to workouts. To find a Personal Day number:

Using March 6 again as a Personal Day:
8 (Personal Year) + 3 (Month) + 6 (Day of the Month)
= 17 1+7 = 8

March 6 becomes an 8 Personal Day, making it an excellent day to add time to workouts.

DOB May 10, 1990
5 + 1 + 0 + 2 + 0 + 1 + 6 = 15 = 1 + 5= 6
Example: Personal Year 6

6 (Personal Year) + 3 (Month) + 6 (Day of the Month)
= 15 1+5 = 6

In a Personal Year 6, it is time to evaluate the current fitness regimen. The focus would be on balancing. Is there balance in your workouts? Is enough time being spent on cardio? Building muscle? How is your flexibility? Do you need to add balancing activities to your workout? Yoga is a good place to start to evaluate this as is an appointment with a good chiropractor. My chiropractor can sum up my fitness in one appointment! She even knows if I am drinking enough water and what excersise and stretches I need to incorporate to create balance in my physical body.

Take a look at the calendar and add your approach to 6 Personal Days which is doing an exercise you love. Go now and add these days to your schedule to amp up your resolve!

CHAPTER 5

How to Prevent Injuries

"Your wealth is in your health."
KELLEY ROSANO

Why do some people have back problems and others never have pain anywhere? How about people who never had a headache, yet others suffer migraines so severe they throw up? The body/mind connection is an interesting one. Often it is attributed to what we *think* are problems. One person's embarrassing trip in an ambulance is another person's Farris wheel ride. Our bodies are prone to different types of weaknesses and susceptible to stress differently because of the way we think about things. Louse Hay has written a fabulous book about the body/mind connection. I encourage you to read *Heal Your Body*, which also includes beautiful affirmations.

While you are in the process of sorting out your thoughts and how they relate to pain and injuries here are some things for you to consider. Soon you will be able to figure these things out for yourself. You will be able to tune into to your body and have a conversation with it just like an old friend. In the meantime take a look at your Health and Wellness Path, so you can start avoiding injuries today. Please copy your Health and Wellness Path number to start your journaling.

Health and Wellness Path 1

Ones tend to be in pain for too long before doing anything about it. This is typical behavior and hopefully after consuming this book, a 1 Path will stop doing such things. Why do you allow this? Are you trying to wish the pain away? Or are you trying to figure out how to fix it yourself? You could, like this writer, succeed in finding ways to remedy the pain on your own and other times you will need to give in and seek a professional. Ones generally have problems in the lower part of the body and later on in life, back problems. The pain will continue until you learn to listen to your body. Pain can come about often and can be attributed to the lack of use. Pushing certain body parts past capacity, then paying the consequences later is how this happens. This will be a cycle for you until you understand that it does not need to be this way.

INJURY/PAIN JOURNALING
PATH 1:

Health and Wellness Path 2

When you want to prevent injuries, pay attention to the way you feel. If you are not feeling up to a task it is best not to do it. You may not use this for an excuse to avoid workouts. If your arms hurt, then walk, do not do push-ups. If your neck hurts, do not use your arms or back. If your legs hurt, do an upper body workout or swim. If you have to do something even though you are not feeling 100% be sure to use positive affirmations. You can tell yourself you will be okay, you will not hurt yourself. "I am strong and fit." "I can do what needs to be done." This is important. You must send love to your body parts when they do not feel well. If you have any healing experience please use this on yourself. You do not need training to send healing and loving thoughts to your body. Use affirmations while holding your mind on the area in pain. Yoga and meditation will help you with this idea.

INJURY/PAIN JOURNALING
PATH 2:

SAY YES TO WHO YOU ARE TO CREATE FITNESS

Health and Wellness Path 3

You need to be creative in order to prevent injuries. The creative ideas you have get jumbled up in your body and mind if you are not expressing them (getting them out by sharing), preventing you from thinking clearly or being able to attend to something fully. This causes your body to get distracted and bad things happen. If you did get hurt playing your favorite game, where was your mind at? Were you jogging and your mind was elsewhere? Then jogging is not a creative enough outlet for you. If you were playing tennis and turned your ankle, maybe you were bored. If you are getting hurt at your job, consider what you were thinking about. When it comes time to do some lifting, like lifting a box, is your mind and body on lifting the box? A mechanic bends down to pick up a tool and hurts their back. Was it the act of bending over or the thoughts in the mind? If a dancer loses focus this could mean disaster. Ask yourself, am I bored? Am I distracted? Or an even better way to look at it is to find engaging enough activities.

INJURY/PAIN JOURNALING
PATH 3:

Health and Wellness Path 4

It is important for fours to realize a plan is needed. Your mind works better if everything is planned. Impromptu things are good, it's the spice of life, but planning can still happen. If a four gets hurt it is most likely a plan was not made for the event occurring. An event like a pick-up basketball game at 5:00 when you have not played in years could end in disaster if a plan is not made. Your body will remember how to play. Run through your mind all things you need to do: warm-up, stretch, cool down. Plan on playing a short time as you have not played in a while. If you have something come up you have never done before, practice a little before you start. Walk through (visualize) the motions in your mind – this will help you so much in everything you do.

INJURY/PAIN JOURNALING
PATH 4:

Health and Wellness Path 5

Variety is the spice of life, fives invented variety. If you are playing a team sport it is best you get a chance to play different positions. This will keep the boredom and injuries at bay. For repetitive movements at work it is beneficial to do opposing motions. Sitting a lot at work requires fives to mix in standing and walking. A very physical job requires frequent opportunities to rest. Most often when fives get hurt it is because they did not take a break from what they were doing. Honoring this is a must, for your five energy can be very intense and life-long injuries can occur if you do not heed your body's needs and tendencies.

INJURY/PAIN JOURNALING
PATH 5:

Health and Wellness Path 6

When a six gets hurt it is related to how they feel about what they are doing. If a six does not really want to be doing an activity, if the heart is not in it, injuries will occur. You can use this to your advantage by considering all the activities you do and have not sustained any injuries. This will be freedom calling! This is related to all aspects of a 6 Paths life. If you get physically hurt, refrain from those activities if possible. Honor the message, for once the injury has occurred, permanent damage could be done. The "I must do this" or "I have to" is fear talking. Most likely there are options you are not considering.

INJURY/PAIN JOURNALING
PATH 6:

Health and Wellness Path 7

If a seven is to avoid injuries, attend to what needs attending. If you are working on arm strength but it is really the legs needing the workout, you risk injury. See, you have a hard time with the truth. The truth will be a leg workout but you will tell yourself to work out your arms. This is also the same for cardio. You will trick yourself into thinking you do not really need it or have done enough. On the other hand, you sevens can over work yourself. Telling yourself, "I need to do more" may also be an untruth. It is best to get an outside opinion. Much of the time if a seven falls victim to an injury, it is self-inflicted. You have allowed an area of your body to become weak by ignoring it. Being able to be a good judge of what you need is possible. It calls for you to sit with it for a while. Ask what area of your body is being ignored. Ask how to best serve your body. Be quiet and see what comes up.

INJURY/PAIN JOURNALING
PATH 7:

Health and Wellness Path 8

If eights want to enjoy a life free of injury, you can. Set the intent. If an eight has reoccurring injuries, look at where the injuries are on the body. This will tell you what is going on. A leg injury: fear of moving forward or making a decision. Arms: fear of what others say or do. Head injury: slow down. You eights are on hyper drive, you see things manifest and want more. You push yourself and cause your own problems. As smart and resourceful as you are, when it comes to slowing down, you really need help. Such evidence should be taken seriously. If you are getting hurt with regularity, you must ask why. You could be asking for signs or answers to questions and it is coming in the form of a physical injury. Eights can manifest, it is their middle name, so those bodily injuries serve as a form of communication.

INJURY/PAIN JOURNALING
PATH 8:

Health and Wellness Path 9

Nines do get injured, not just in the line of duty but you often get injured when you need to accomplish something in short order. You resent being pushed, even if it is your own doing. It is best not to rush anything, be it work or play. Use your sense of time to your advantage and make sure you have enough time to do each task. You are just asking for trouble if you do not honor this in yourself. You can make magic with a few resources but time is something else. Time is a resource which is rather solid. Some projects or fitness goals are time sensitive, that's just how life is, plan accordingly.

INJURY/PAIN JOURNALING
PATH 9:

CHAPTER 6

How to Support Yourself

"The Angels don't take offense if we keep
asking over and over again."
DOREEN VIRTUE

It is imperative you start your next step toward wellness as soon as possible. When you leave that gap of time in there, too many things can happen to confirm *now* is not the right time. There is no better time to start taking better care of yourself then right now.

If it is motivation you lack, here are some positive affirmations to get you started. If you only take one step toward wellness, this would be it. Upon waking each morning, write or recite reasons you want a healthy life, reasons you want to be fit, or benefits you will get from this new approach. Reading affirmations is good but actively creating your own statements is better.

- ♥ I am healthy and have energy all day.
- ♥ I can create all my dreams and goals to become the picture of health.
- ♥ It is in my own best interest to be fit and healthy.
- ♥ I love to eat right and exercise every day.
- ♥ I have the will power it takes to make these changes in my life.
- ♥ I trust myself to make good decisions.
- ♥ Good morning, sexy new you, let's go kick some ass!
- ♥ Let's walk with Spirit today and say hi to the angels.
- ♥ I eat what I need and listen to my body.

Now, pause for a moment. Did you make your own statements while reading this? Quick, write them down before you forget. Make a copy of this journal page.

POSITIVE AFFIRMATION JOURNALING:

- ♥
- ♥
- ♥
- ♥
- ♥
- ♥
- ♥
- ♥
- ♥
- ♥
- ♥
- ♥
- ♥
- ♥

Be sure none of your statements are at the detriment of someone else. You can always add "this or something better" onto any statement. Each one of your affirmations will have a special blessing with the energy of this book. The blessings you get with your intentions to improve your health with be three fold. It is good to recognize the power of intent. I have the power of intent to bless you. My guides offer their blessings, as well as all my angels. This special blessing will support you. Reread this section each time you feel you need extra support and know you can call upon any angel or guide to assist you in your path to wellness. They want to help- they really do.

Archangel Raphael wants to heal all the aspects of our lives which create chaos in our bodies. Call on Archangel Raphael to heal anything you feel is impeding your progress.

Call on *Archangel Gabriel* when you need a push in your workouts. She wants you to feel physically strong and competent. You will find much more ease of mind when your body is physically fit.

When you are in need of making the best dietary choices call on *Archangel Michael.* He wants you to nourish your body to the fullest capacity, knowing you will need your energy to fulfill your life purpose.

In the event you are in a bind and cannot do anything on your list for the day, call on *Archangel Jophiel* to uplift you so you can make it to the next best option. She will be sure your choice is the best for you in your circumstances.

If organization or writing things down is a block to your success call upon *Medatron.* He will assist you in getting and staying organized. His energy is nervousness, so the next time you 'feel' a little nervous, tune in and see what *Medatron* is trying to communicate.

Archangel Raguel is 2 energy. When you need cooperation and balance ask him for help. Keeping the color of light blue near or around you will be a calling card to him when you need his support. Paint your new studio a pleasing shade of light blue if you want to add fitness to your life every day.

When clearing is needed or to release what does not serve you, *Archangel Zadkiel* is here for the job. He wants you to let go of things easily so he will guide you on the path of least resistance.

Make a copy of this page to journal on your Archangel connections:

ARCHANGEL JOURNALING:

Date	Angel	Notes

Know whichever Archangel you call upon, you cannot make a mistake. They all will help you in caring for your body. Also, know whenever you make an attempt to get in better health, your body hears you. Your body knows you are trying. If the feeling of failure comes over you, you need to do all you can to stop it from continuing. This is like fire to your resolve. You must make every attempt to change your mood. Even at the cost of relationships. It could be people causing you to have a hard time. Those people need to go or be set aside. Soon, you will be able to block them out but in the beginning you will need all the help you can get.

If you need to be sure this program will work for you, take a few moments to consider how things are going for you right now. If you could change just one thing, right now, what would it be? Now glance at the book and see if the answer/approach is here. My guess it is. It is the law. The Law of Attraction. If, in the event you are disappointed with what you find here after asking yourself this question, give it 24 hours. If after this amount time has gone by and you truly cannot see yourself doing anything in this book, by all means pass it on.

When it is necessary to make changes, most often it is best they are not made under duress. You can expect crazy things to happen when you make choices from this perspective. Desperation and the 'gatta do something now' energy will not work, no matter what information you find.

Much of my work is about soul searching. This is important. When you take the time to explore and get to know who you are, many of the bells and whistles stop going off. Feelings of desperation cause the bells and whistles. Similarly to how electrons act differently when someone is observing them. When your body knows you are paying attention and you want to make decisions for the greater good, it will respond.

Here are some positive attributes about yourself for you to include in the affirmations you create. I put it in list form. You can grab out the ones you like the most about yourself. It is also important to include attributes about yourself which seem really far from your truth. Remember an emotional reaction to the words is what you are looking for. There is space provided next to your word list to write your affirmations. Make a photocopy of this page before you begin or if this is not your book, please get another piece of paper for your notes. Good luck and have fun with these.

POSITIVE AFFIRMATION JOURNALING:

Health and Wellness Path 1

Unique
Genuine
Leader
Innovative
Benevolent
Creativity

POSITIVE AFFIRMATION JOURNALING:

Health and Wellness Path 2

Sensitive
Body Awareness
Balanced
Cooperative
Romantic
Caring

POSITIVE AFFIRMATION JOURNALING:

Health and Wellness Path 3

Creative
Visionary
Joy
Expressive
Initiative
Adaptable

POSITIVE AFFIRMATION JOURNALING:

Health and Wellness Path 4

Organized
Reliable
Systematic
Focused
Thoughtful
Solid

POSITIVE AFFIRMATION JOURNALING:

Health and Wellness Path 5

Flexible
Curious
Variety
Movement
Tolerant
Expansive

POSITIVE AFFIRMATION JOURNALING:

Health and Wellness Path 6

Unconditional
Nurturer
Domestic
Perfectionist
Beauty
Intuition

POSITIVE AFFIRMATION JOURNALING:

Health and Wellness Path 7

Truth
Knowledge
Objective
Open
Bridge
Wisdom

POSITIVE AFFIRMATION JOURNALING:

Health and Wellness Path 8

Power
Abundance
Orchestrator
Makes Things Happen
Justice
Ambitious

POSITIVE AFFIRMATION JOURNALING:

Health and Wellness Path 9

Humanitarian
Empower
Compassionate
Talented
Inspiring
Fun

When you consider all you have been through to get to the point you are now, is it really hard to imagine things will get better? It is from my experience I tell you things will get better. Your intent is the power you need. If you sabotage your intent or allow others to sabotage it, this is another matter. The above affirmations will help you stay the course. You can begin to see all you intend will come to light. Yes, it does take some effort but not the kind you think. Replace the word effort with "awareness". It only takes awareness. Not having a good day, takes awareness. You need not have a complete breakdown because of it. There were many times before when you had a bad day and did not even notice but proceeded to eat half a tray of brownies or skip your workout. Funny how a different perspective makes all the difference. Now, when you have a 'not so great day,' you can focus on the fact you noticed. When you notice, now have the tool to help you turn it into a better day.

With Love and Light and many Blessings on each page, Tricia

www.ingramcontent.com/pod-product-compliance
Lightning Source LLC
Chambersburg PA
CBHW020518290526
45786CB00002B/655